HOMEOPATHY
HIPPOCRATIC MEDICINE
MO MORRISH

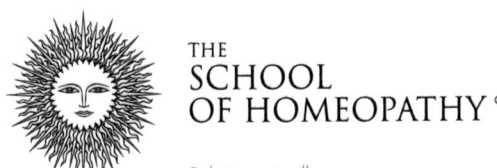

Be better, naturally...

Published in the UK by The School of Homeopathy
An imprint of In-Light
Orchard Leigh · Rodborough Hill
Stroud · Gloucestershire · GL5 3SS

First published: 2020
Website: www.schoolofhomeopathy.com
Email: info@soh.uk.com
© School of Homeopathy

ISBN: 978-0-9544766-5-6

Written by Mo Morrish
Edited by Brian Turpin
Design and typesetting by Mani Norland
Printed and bound in the UK

British Library Cataloguing in Publishing Data. A catalogue record for this book is available from the British Library.

All rights reserved. No part of this publication may be stored in a retrieval system, transmitted or reproduced in any way, including but not limited to photocopy, photograph, magnetic or other record, without prior agreement and written permission of the author.

This book contains general information only. The author accepts no liability for injury, loss or damage to anyone acting on the contents of this book. No responsibility is accepted for any errors or omissions in the contents of the book.

DEDICATION

This is respectfully dedicated to the millions of people all around the world who have benefited from homeopathic treatment. You made your own experience so you know how effective homeopathy can be.

CONTENTS

Foreword	8
Statement	11
Introduction	13
Health	16
Sickness	19
Help	20
Harm	22
The World	24
The Human	26
The Individual	30
Susceptibility	32
Science and Art	35
Hahnemann	37
The Unprejudiced Observer	39
The Principles	40
The Potencies	45
The Provings	48

The Practice	51
How does it Work?	58
Evidence	62
Scientists	66
Scrutiny	71
Homeopaths	74
Homeopathy	76
Homeopathy and the NHS	78
Unifying Medicine	82
References	84
Further Reading	87
Acknowledgements	88

FOREWORD
DR MICHAEL DIXON LVO, OBE, MA, FRCGP, FRCC

This book is an excellent description and defence of homeopathy. It is pithy, elegantly written and argued with integrity. It is also a great read with wonderful quotes.

I see it as a plea for personalised medicine rather than simply the application of population-based evidence. Good medicine needs to include both. As the author says, we must not polarise between Western medicine and complementary medicine as both have their place or, in his words "both approaches are helpful". I also see this book as a plea for a form of medicine that goes with the grain of nature and nudges our own natural processes of healing and health. Conventional medicine, which has been so effective in so many ways with diseases such as cancer and heart attacks often works by challenging and reversing nature's processes. Again, there is room for both perspectives but wherever possible there is a strong case - in terms of safety and sustained effectiveness as well as a human and economic case – for supporting rather than confronting the forces of nature.

I am not a homeopath but simply an observer. What I do observe is that many of my patients are being helped by homeopaths. I observe consultations that are often more personal and have more depth than I am able to offer in the standard ten-minute NHS consultation. I also observe my own profession feeling threatened and defensive in the face of a model of healing that they cannot understand or explain. I also observe that when it comes to research, we are too often asking the wrong questions and getting the wrong answers. As a pragmatic GP, I am not too concerned as to whether a patient's recovery is due to the medication, his own characteristics, those of the therapist or, indeed, the interaction between them. What I really want to know is something along the lines of "if a patient has headaches, irritable bowel or a sense of hopelessness, for instance, which treatment is more effective – conventional treatment or seeing a homeopath?" In too many areas, we don't have the answers and the much-needed research has not been funded by an NHS that unfairly spends 0% of its research budget on complementary medicine. Covid has changed everything. We are now living in a time of uncertainty when we need to view the world with new eyes. In this new world I think we will regard it as strange that an NHS that spent £127 billion in 2016 felt it appropriate to cut its relatively tiny budget of £92,000 on homeopathy. It was an act of meanness supported by some over vociferous clinicians, scientists and senior managers. But in the end, it doesn't matter what any of them think - it is the patients that matter. They are quite rightly the focus of this book, which I see as a healing of the divide between the conventional and the complementary. In a pluralist society, we must keep our minds and hearts open and I believe that this book will be helpful to patients, therapists and clinicians of every kind.

STATEMENT

My experience is this: Through thirty years of homeopathic practise I have helped several thousand people restore themselves to health, or to significantly improve their health, without causing any harm. I consider this to be a reasonable, ethical, honest and helpful way to earn a modest living chiming, as it does, with the Hippocratic dictum of:
"Either help, or at least do no harm".

INTRODUCTION

In 2020 Britain, as in much of the world, almost every aspect of healthcare is in crisis. We struggle collectively with increasing levels of depression and anxiety, obesity and diabetes, and allergies of all kinds. Meanwhile, chronic conditions such as heart disease, cancer, asthma, eczema, migraine, menstrual disorders, arthritis etc. continue to be ever-present and all set against a back-drop of looming antimicrobial resistance. Whilst many more of us live longer, an increasing number of us take more and more drugs suggesting that we are not as healthy as we may think.

In addition, post the Covid-19 pandemic, we anticipate an increase in people with mental health issues and post-viral fatigue as well as the suffering of the many people whose cancer treatments were delayed. It seems timely for a collective pause within which to reconsider and re-evaluate the wide range of healing modalities available to us. Alongside mainstream medicine, these include homeopathy, osteopathy, chiropractic, herbalism, acupuncture, psychotherapy, nutrition and many others. If we were more informed about these healing tools, we would make much more appropriate health choices for ourselves and our families. This would also benefit the NHS which, especially since its pandemic heroics, is struggling to meet all the demands made upon it.

This book has been written for all those who are open to a wider consideration of medicine, how to help more yet cause less harm. It represents a distillation of thirty years of homeopathic practice and much reflection upon that experience as well as the works of, amongst many others, Hippocrates, Samuel Hahnemann, Albert Einstein, and Lao Tsu. Each of these has based their work upon unprejudiced observation and experiment, filtered through intelligent and insightful minds. Not one of them was afraid to challenge accepted authority. The title of this little book alludes to the consistent observation made by the "father of medicine" over two and a half thousand years ago, that there is more than one approach to healing and we would be wise to embrace them. While he wrote about the use of herbs, exercise and nutrition, he pointedly drew attention to the notion of healing with both opposites and similars. As will be explained later, my proposal is that these two terms apply to modern mainstream medicine and homeopathy, respectively. Samuel Hahnemann experimented tirelessly and evolved the system of homeopathy which is described here, and Einstein is quoted here as that rare scientist who applied both left and right brain function to an exploration of the universe agreeing as it does with Lao Tsu's observation that seeming opposites actually complement one another.

This is a little book by design; it is intended to be minimalist, succinct and clear so that any discussion of the ideas presented at least begins with clarity. My aim is to present homeopathy as a valid and important modality within a unified field of medicine. You do not have to agree with or believe in anything written here, I only hope that you are encouraged to keep your mind open.

You are also encouraged to notice how you are reading this little book. With an open mind, or one closed and already decided.

HEALTH

We can regard health as the optimum expression of the individual, mentally, emotionally, physically, socially and spiritually (whatever that means to the person) with the least friction with his or her environment.

Each individual is a unique expression of Life and so health is a dynamic state, subject to change, which must be considered relative to states which preceded it, and relative to other members of the collective.

The environment here refers to those factors which influence each person in a positive or negative manner. Examples include the dynamics of familial and personal relationships, beliefs and thinking patterns, work, housing, and nourishment on all levels as well as cultural, ideological, geographical and global elements. As is well documented, social and financial inequality impact hugely on the health of millions of people while the Earth, heavily-populated and polluted by humans, is facing a climate catastrophe and many cultures are in states of turmoil, riven as they are by all the "isms" of divisiveness (the insistence of one way over another).

The quality of health is ease and freedom; freedom from constriction, resistance and pain.

The health of the collective, the community or nation, can be considered in a similar way; the optimum expression of the general population, mentally, emotionally, physically, socially and spiritually, with the least friction with the shared environment. More and more people are suffering on all these levels as evidenced by the well documented crises in mental health, in epidemics of obesity and loneliness, in increased sensitivities to the external environment such as allergies, food intolerances and asthma.

In 2014, following a 70% increase in prescription drugs over a decade, the NHS reported that almost half of all adults take prescription drugs (an average of 18.7 prescriptions per head of the population in one year)[1] and that in 2016 there were 64.7 million prescriptions for anti-depressants in England, more than double the previous decade, which then had a population of 54.79 million people.[2] Whilst we are living longer, we apparently need more and more medication. Healthy people, surely, don't need medication.

Good health is the best defence against invading bacteria and viruses.

When I was a secondary schoolboy in the mid 60s, there was one boy in the whole school who had a chronic disease whose name no one was sure of pronouncing correctly; asthma.

Nowadays most teachers have a drawer stuffed with inhalers. What has happened to the health of our people, and why? Why are these questions not being asked of governments, health services and the pharmaceutical industry?

"Health is the greatest of human blessings."

Hippocrates

Instead of simply considering health, we could take a more rounded view and also consider well-being. Well-being is not the same as health. Well-being suggests a successful acceptance of, and adaptation to, one's situation. Example: "I am managing my disease as best I can and am enjoying life, and expressing myself as fully as possible, within the limits imposed upon me."

The quality is a feeling of contentment or comfort.

SICKNESS

Sickness is the other side of the coin to health in that one state cannot exist without its polar opposite; they arise mutually and may be viewed as relative states of ease. We can regard sickness as the inhibited expression of the individual on any level, mental, emotional, physical, social and spiritual, often due to friction with his/her environment.

The quality of sickness is unease, restriction and pain.

Regarding sickness, Hippocrates suggested that: **"There are no diseases, only sick people"**. Whilst we can all agree that, "this is a case of influenza or cholera", he is reminding us that the disease does not exist on its own, that the "case" is a susceptible human being. He goes further by suggesting that: **"It is more important to know the person who has the condition than it is to know the condition the person has"**. Whilst it is important to have knowledge of both the condition and the person, it also makes sense to consider the patient as an individual, for that is what she/he undoubtedly is.

As Hippocrates also stated so succinctly: **"In the case of disease make a habit of two things; either help, or at least do no harm."**

HELP

To help in this context is to make it easier for the patient to continue in life, or towards peaceful death; to ease suffering and pain; to assist the patient towards ease. The first thing for any helper is to be fully present to the needs of the patient. Even in extremis, a connection between them can make a difference to the outcome; a look, a smile, a touch.

"Some patients, though conscious that their condition is perilous, recover their health simply through their contentment with the goodness of the physician."

Hippocrates

The primary qualities of any helper then are attentive presence, empathy and simple kindness. These qualities, allied with knowledge, expertise and experience, are what all patients hope for.

Painkillers and steroids, for example, can be helpful; simple listening to someone in distress can be helpful; first aid is generally very helpful. Even so, Hahnemann is clear that the **"physician's high and only mission is to restore the sick to health"**.

This suggests more, much more, than simply managing the symptoms (although such palliation may be all that is possible) but involves the full restoration of health, a restoration which, ideally, is rapid, gentle and permanent. This in turn suggests that whatever is causing the symptoms needs to be fully resolved. As an example, the simple removal of a tumour without an attempt to address the process which gave rise to it can only be palliation. This situation is comparable to the removal of the bulb when a warning light flashes on your car's dashboard.

A treatment or medicine which eases symptoms is helpful; a treatment or medicine which resolves the cause of the symptoms is much more helpful. A continuation of helpfulness is to teach the patient how to avoid those things which cause illness; essentially a raising of awareness around lifestyle choices and general preventative measures.

"The greatest medicine of all is teaching people not to need it".
Hippocrates

As helpful as modern mainstream medicine can be, it is not the only way to help relieve suffering. Millions of people continue to derive great health benefit from homoeopathy, herbalism, acupuncture, chiropractic, osteopathy, psychotherapy, therapeutic massage, and many other treatment modalities. Whether or not you believe they are placebo, have an evidence base or an explainable mechanism, they help.

HARM

Most medical practitioners, of any modality, do not set out to cause additional harm, injury, distress or suffering to their patients. None-the-less, harm is caused and iatrogenesis is the term for such harm; "caused by the doctor"/practitioner. Harm may be caused in a number of different ways; negligence, ignorance, human error, nocebo (opposite to placebo) nosocomial infections (hospital acquired) invasive diagnostic procedures, un-necessary surgery and, most commonly, adverse drug reactions.

Whilst not listed by the CDC (Centers for Disease Control and Prevention) there is sound evidence to suggest that iatrogenesis is the third leading cause of death in both the USA and the UK, behind heart disease and cancer. This is likely to be more associated with the influence of the pharmaceutical industry than the medical profession.[3]

Jeremy Hunt MP, a previous serving Minister for Health said in an interview with the Observer in 2020, that the biggest surprise he encountered in the role was finding out that "150 people a week die in the NHS because of errors in their medical treatment. I was gobsmacked by that. Then I discovered this was actually true all over the world; this is what happens in medicine."[4]

Whilst this is alarming, it is not my intention here to point any blame at the medical profession; helping people can be an uncertain and risky business and some treatments simply do not give the desired result. I have enormous respect for the doctors and nurses worldwide who do their utmost to help, often under increasingly difficult conditions (including the pressures of litigation). Even so, with the very best will in the world, modern mainstream medicine both helps, and causes harm.

In the interests of balance, it needs to be stated that mainstream medicine helps such a phenomenal number of people that gathering statistics is impossible. It provides the best emergency treatment on Earth and the positive impact of surgery can be almost miraculous. It is in the area of chronic illness that the mainstream approach has serious limitations, depending, as it does, upon the often-continuous prescription of drugs.

THE WORLD

Before a consideration of Homeopathy itself, I offer a world view within which to frame that consideration.

It is generally agreed amongst scientists that the universe began around 13.8 billion years ago when a tiny point of infinite heat and density, smaller than an atomic nucleus, emerged out of seeming nothing. Within a trillion trillionth of a second this "singularity" expanded with incomprehensible speed to astronomical size, and is still expanding. Time and space immediately arose and matter emerged from energy; as time passed and matter cooled, diverse kinds of atoms began to form and eventually condensed into our universe.

Put very simply; something (the singularity) emerged from seeming nothing, or mystery, and this gave rise to everything. When something emerged from nothing, polarity came into existence. "This" emerged from "that", "is" from "is not"; matter emerged from energy (the basic "stuff" of which the universe is made which, when extremely intense, forms matter) and a multitude of complementary pairs of opposites came into being, each giving rise to the other. Examples include *chaos* and *order*, *light* and *dark*, *expansion* and *contraction*, *hot* and *cold*, *unknown* and *known*, *alive* and *dead*, *active* and *passive*, *masculine* and *feminine*, *love* and *hate* (the list is endless).

Western thought has always favoured one pole over the other, pitted one against the other; *good* against *bad*, *positive* against *negative*, *male* over *female*. This contributes to a linear mode of thought rather than a cyclical one and unless challenged, tends to lead towards the notion of progress. It is just not possible to have one pole without the other; *north* without *south*, for example, or *self* without *other*, *poverty* without *wealth*, *sickness* without *health*, *absence* without *presence*; batteries need *positive* and *negative* poles, computers need the *on* and *off* of the binary coding. Attempting to eradicate one pole is futile and threatens the whole.

Perhaps the most insidious example arises from the delusion that we humans are separate from Nature, while the reality is that we are of Nature, as much as any species. This division between *us* and *the world* easily leads on to unhelpful narratives such as "*us* and *them*", promoting divide at the expense of unite, *exclude* at the expense of *include* and so allowing our species to take what it wants from the whole, the Earth and all other life forms, without any thought of consequences. Current politics and much of the media are examples of the toxicity which stems from such divisiveness.

What is real is that we live in a polarized universe composed essentially of energy (in various forms, including matter) and subject to constant change; every action is followed, sooner or later, by reaction. We know this to be so yet we act as if we don't know; this is likely to limit our thinking, to narrow our "mindedness".

THE HUMAN

All medical practitioners of all persuasions would, I am sure, agree that the patient is made up of tangible elements, less tangible elements and those that are intangible. The bones, tissues and organs, for example, are clearly visible to the naked eye, have weight and dimension. Less tangible aspects include the endocrine system, through which tiny amounts of hormone are released at often unpredictable times with striking effect. Or the nervous system through which electrical impulses leap across microscopic gaps (synapses) and billions of intercranial neurons interact to allow thinking and experience. The immune system is apparently everywhere within the body but is not everywhere obvious. Intangibles include consciousness, and Life itself.

I find it incredibly helpful to remind myself, often, that the human is a self-regulating, self-creating organism composed of trillions of cells all functioning together in harmonious vital process. It has evolved over two million years and, whilst obviously needing assistance at times, is a pretty robust, self-healing phenomenon.

Apparently, around seven billion, billion, billion atoms come together to form me, an average human adult, and it has been estimated that in one year's time 98% of those atoms will have been replaced, and yet today I will still remember my third birthday party, and be recognized as me. Isn't that amazing!

How does that everyday miracle occur? The answer, as far as we can attempt one, is complex but it seems reasonable to suggest that there is some kind of organizing principle at work, some invisible and intangible element which organizes me as me and maintains homeostasis while I watch television or sleep. My body/mind performs a literally unquantifiable number of tasks, including the exchange of material, energy and information with my environment, without my being remotely aware. Through the complex processes of building up and breaking down (anabolism and catabolism) this organizing principle seems to conduct the continuous re-composing of me, maintaining sensation and function which is normal to me. When my personal organizer is disturbed I may experience changes in my normal sensation and function, which we call symptoms, and in my general state, which we term sickness. If my personal organizer is broken beyond repair or leaves, then I will die and instead of recomposing I will decompose. When death comes, when there is no more animation of the seven billion, billion, billion atoms, there is no doubt about it, it is apparent to all.

A simpler example of an organizing principle can be observed in the snowflake. It is commonly known that no two snowflakes are alike but if they are photographed, melted, re-frozen and then photographed again they appear exactly as before as if the water molecules arranged themselves upon an invisible template of some kind.

From this way of seeing things, disease is seen as a disturbance in the organism and symptoms are an *expression* of that. From the more general perspective of modern mainstream medicine, symptoms are seen as the disease. It is clear that in order to fully cure the patient it is necessary to consider what disturbed her/him and in what manner the disturbance is being expressed.

Thus, there would appear to be two essential approaches to this attempt at cure. Either treat the symptoms alone, in which case drugs which induce the opposite effect are useful e.g. treat inflammation with an anti-inflammatory, depression with an anti-depressant etc. Or, through a careful consideration of the symptoms and the factors which gave rise to them, treat the disturbance itself. As a disturbance is a state and more complex than a single symptom of it, treating with opposites is not likely to prove successful. What, after all, is the opposite of influenza or shock? The most helpful relationship between the medicine and the disease from this point of view would seem to be that of similarity i.e. a medicine which in trials on healthy people induces a symptom complex or state which is very similar to that observed in the patient.

In very simple terms, modern medicine attempts to fight *against* disease from a Western perspective, adopting a somewhat pugilistic approach; homeopathy, on the other hand, works *with* the organizing principle, in the manner of the martial arts such as Ju-jitsu or Aikido. **Both** approaches are helpful.

My suggestion is that we lessen the polarizing and divisive attitude of *either/or* and increase the unifying and inclusive attitude of *and/both*, depending on what the patient needs in the moment.

From the above perspective, disease is regarded as a dynamic disturbance of the whole person. Symptoms may be produced anywhere within the body-mind yet the entire self-regulating organism is dis-eased, not just a part. Even a disturbance as simple and physical as stepping on a nail will elicit symptoms on several levels: pain, anger, negative thoughts ("I might get infected and die!") It makes sense to treat the person from a holistic perspective; in fact, my suggestion is that this is the only way to treat.

THE INDIVIDUAL

That each human being is unique is an un-assailable fact of biology. Whilst each of us is 99.9% genetically identical, we each come into this life with our own particular mix of parental genes and epi-genetic variations which, together, we might term our basic constitution or make-up; this corresponds to "nature". Then things happen to us and these experiences further shape the person we are constantly becoming; "nurture/non-nurture".

Human being is an activity which is constant until we die. We each attract certain influences and react to them according to our individual make-up and inherited and acquired susceptibilities, or sensitivities. When disturbed or "dis-eased", we each express this in our own way.

When examining a patient there are three aspects to consider:

- **The appearance**
- bleeding, shortness of breath, pallor, perspiration, trembling etc. This would also include objective signs which can be read, such as laboratory test results, X-rays, MRI scans etc.
- **The condition:** essentially, the symptoms as experienced by the patient.
- **The state:** characterized by the behavior.

Example 1: A man in a hospital ward suffering with pneumonia. He has a very ruddy complexion, lies very still with his back to everyone, and periodically sits up to drink an entire glass of cold water. Groaning, he lies back down again and when the nurse asks if he is alright, he curtly tells her to leave him alone.

Example 2: Another man in a hospital bed suffering with pneumonia. He is sitting up in bed with three pillows and sipping from a glass of cold water. He is pale, well groomed, wears an immaculate silk dressing gown and holds onto the nurse's hand, with his trembling hand, because he does not want to be left alone.

Both men are suffering with pneumonia and both men have been prescribed the same antibiotic, which may or may not be helpful. They are each in a different disease state, each expressing 'pneumonia' in an individual way, each needing a different medicine, corresponding to that state.

SUSCEPTIBILITY

Susceptibility is fundamental to the practice of any medical approach. It implies a tendency or open-ness to being influenced by something external, such as a virus. Within a medical context, the immune system of the patient yields to the influence and symptoms are induced; the patient is sick.

The range and intensity of these symptoms is dependent upon the degree to which the person yields. Some people are only slightly open to the viral influence and so produce only mild symptoms such as a slightly raised temperature and a dry cough. Others may be highly susceptible, so open to the malign influence that they may suffer life threatening symptoms such as severe, acute respiratory or pulmonary distress. There are also some people who are not at all open to the viral influence; they are immune to it and may be symptom-less carriers.

At a certain point in the process of being influenced, or infected, the immune system of the patient responds, or reacts. This response may be inadequate, resulting in continuing sickness or death; adequate, resulting in recovery and potential future immunity; or excessive, an allergic reaction.

Susceptibility is an individual quality based upon genetic, epi-genetic, and constitutional factors ("nature") as well as life-style and life-story factors ("nurture/non-nurture"). My suggestion is that susceptibility and reaction (opposite poles of the same phenomenon, sensitivity, which can also be expressed through the complementary pair, yield and respond) together give a good idea of what a person is sensitive to, how that sensitivity is expressed and to what degree. For example, a person sensitive to a peanut, produces a rapid swelling of the bronchi and goes into anaphylactic shock.

It rationally follows that the cure of any disease must, surely, address both the underlying susceptibility of a patient to a particular influence and also their reaction to that influence. The best treatment, therefore, will be one that is specific for each individual. Cure also involves the susceptibility of the patient to the medicine; whether it will help, do nothing, or cause harm.

As a young bacteriologist I was inculcated with the "Germ Theory" of disease, as put forward by Pasteur (the "father of bacteriology") and Koch. Stated simply, micro-organisms cause disease. Yet many people did not die in any given epidemic or pandemic; why not? Because they were not susceptible. Before he died Pasteur changed his approach insisting that it was less to do with the microbe and more to do with the terrain, the susceptibility of the individual.

Germ theory and Terrain theory *together* allow a consideration of the whole. The greater the degree of health, the less the susceptibility to invading micro-organisms such as viruses and bacteria. Homeopathy stimulates the patient as a whole, increasing the health and resilience and thus decreasing susceptibility to infectious disease processes.

SCIENCE AND ART

"The most beautiful experience we can have is the mysterious. It is the source of all true art and science".

Einstein

The greater part of the universe is the unknown, the mysterious. As humans, we cannot help but explore this. Our polarised, bi-lobed brain offers us two opposing ways to explore; left brain, logical, objective, reductive (science) and right brain, intuitive, subjective, holistic (art). Both sides interact, complement and complete one another. For example; the left brain is credited with language, yet the right brain provides context and tone. To avoid narrow-mindedness, we need both.

Science is an incredibly useful tool, a method for exploring the universe which continues to exert a profound effect upon all our lives, witness the extraordinary technology available to us now. It is a methodology in which objectivity is valued at the expense of subjective experience, yet each scientist brings his or her subjective or emotional selves to the experiment; his or her conscious or unconscious prejudices. It is not the only way to explore and make sense of the world. Art may be seen as the reflection upon, and expression of, the subjective experience of both individuals and collectives which also helps us to explore and make sense of the world. Of itself, science cannot determine whether something is beautiful, meaningful, musical or funny: only a human being can do that, by using faculties other than logic. Equally, art does not help us solve problems of food production, transportation, communication or surgery. We need both.

Einstein suggested that: *"It would be possible to describe everything scientifically, but it would make no sense; it would be without meaning, as if you described a Beethoven symphony as a variation of wave pressure"*.

A similar expression of the science/art dynamic has been the apparent conflict between science and religion (see "The God Delusion", Richard Dawkins and "The Science Delusion", Rupert Sheldrake). Einstein, that physicist who understood the unity behind duality, succinctly brought the two together: *"Science without religion is lame; religion without science is blind"*.

And, commenting on science alone: *"One thing I have learned in a long life: that all our science, measured against reality is primitive and child-like, and yet it is the most precious thing we have."*

HAHNEMANN

As Hippocrates is known as the father of medicine, so Samuel Hahnemann is the father of homeopathy; he established the fundamental principles of this science and art, based upon careful observation and experiment.

Born in Germany in 1755, Hahnemann became fluent in six or seven languages and qualified as a physician at a young age. After some time, he realized that the treatments of the day were causing more harm than good; he could not comply with the Hippocratic dictum, so he gave up the practice of medicine and earned a living for his family by translating pharmacological textbooks. In one, he read that Cinchona bark was a cure for malaria because, "it had a bitter effect upon the stomach". Being a thinker, he knew that many things had such an effect so, in a well described experiment published in a journal of the time, he ingested some Cinchona bark. Shortly afterwards, he became ill and, once he had recovered, noticed that the symptoms he had experienced were very similar to those of malarial patients; it was as if he had suffered malaria. He wondered if this might be an expression of a healing principle, that a substance which induced symptoms in a healthy person similar to those in the sick person might, somehow, be medicinal.

Hahnemann then experimented on close to two hundred substances, tested in trials on healthy people, and thus created the beginning of a pharmacy which has since grown to around two thousand medicines. These trials are called "provings" from the German word, "pruefung" which means "to test". The homeopathic pharmacy is known as the "Materia Medica".

Hahnemann also described the primary and secondary actions of medicines, introduced the concept of epigenetics (which he called "miasms") called for an evidence base for the popular treatment of blood-letting, called for a more humane approach to the treatment of patients suffering with their mental health, and recognized the impact of poor hygiene on the proliferation of disease.

Hahnemann was a prolific experimenter and writer. He revised his "Organon of the Medical Art" six times; wrote a stunning work of epidemiology in 1838, "The Chronic Diseases"; and collected the exact symptoms induced by the provings in his "Materia Medica Pura".

Hahnemann has been airbrushed from the history of medicine.

THE UNPREJUDICED OBSERVER

Hahnemann introduced the concept of the unprejudiced observer to medicine. Given that each patient is truly an individual and therefore requires a medicine which resonates with that individuality, it is quite clear that each patient must be explored as a never previously observed phenomenon. This requires that the healer makes no assumptions and does not pre-judge the patient, the treatment or the outcome.

"A man should look for what is, and not for what he thinks should be".

Einstein

My suggestion is that a true scientist is an unprejudiced observer, someone who sees things as they are, not as they are supposed to be or expected to be. Whilst it is understood that it is **"harder to crack prejudice than an atom"** (Einstein) a true scientist and a homeopath will do their utmost to be as pure in their observations as they can.

THE PRINCIPLES

Homeopathy: the word is derived from the Greek and means "similar suffering". To prescribe homeopathically means to prescribe a medicine which, in trials on healthy people, induces a similar symptom complex or dis-eased state to that observed in the patient. At first, this may seem a little counterintuitive so a few examples may help to clarify this first principle. In a typical case of childhood illness, the patient often presents as if he/she had eaten Belladonna berries found near the allotment or country garden; symptoms would commonly include dilated pupils, flushed face, throbbing carotids, high temperature and a restless delirium. Belladonna, given in homeopathic potency, has been found to be very helpful; an observation which has been made continuously over nearly two hundred years.

It seems that the poison, when prepared in the homeopathic manner, becomes the medicine. This has echoes in the old expression, "Take the hair of the dog that bit you".

If we were to take you into the desert for three to four hours with no shade or water and then bring you into a Bedouin tent for relief, which would restore you quickest and best; a glass of cold water or a glass of hot tea? Although it appears to run counter to common sense, the best medicine would be the hot tea. You are suffering from heat so the first aid part of treatment is to remove you from the cause, and to then give you the hot liquid. In a similar way, agricultural workers toiling in the midday sun would be best served to get into some shade and drink a small amount of a warming liquid such as brandy or red wine, and then, gradually, cool water to rehydrate.

When little children play in the snow, they seem to always lose at least one glove and then begin to cry with the pain of cold hands. Once back indoors the child instinctively wants to put its hands close to a source of heat. The blood vessels have constricted; if strong heat is introduced then the blood vessels will dilate too quickly and that will induce pain also (which increases again when the hands are taken away from the heat source). The best treatment is a gentle application of cool followed by warm; not strong heat. Action is followed by reaction and a strong action is followed by a strong counteraction.

A medicine which induces a similar symptom complex as that observed in the patient is likely to resonate with the organizing principle of the patient which has, after all, produced symptoms that are similar to those of the prover/tester. To put this another way, the self-regulating organism, the patient, is likely to be susceptible to a medicine which induces similar symptoms in other human beings.

Similarity suggests resonance.

The most well-known example of the homoeopathic principle of "similar" is, of course, vaccination. A small, attenuated dose of something which causes a certain disease is given to prevent the same or similar disease. Edward Jenner and his use of Cowpox vesicles to prevent Smallpox is the original and much celebrated example. Also, the current conventional treatment of allergies and hypersensitivity involves the use of tiny amounts of the offending allergen.

The homeopathicity of vaccination is compromised by the addition of chemical preservatives to the similar material. These have their own particular effects upon susceptible people.

The second principle of homeopathy is to prescribe one medicine at a time; this is simple science, good sense and both understood and appreciated by homeopathic patients worldwide. If changes occur after any single medical intervention it is reasonable to suppose that those changes, positive or negative, are likely to have arisen because of the intervention; this means that the practitioner has some idea of what is happening within the patient, what direction things are going in and what is the most sensible way forward. If more than one medical stimulus is applied at the same time it becomes increasingly difficult for any practitioner to know what is happening or what to do next. As an example, Age UK has recently reported that around 20 percent of recently retired people are taking an average of five pharmaceutical drugs a day—and by the time they reach the age of 85, this will have risen to eight drugs.[5] These drugs are not trialled together and individual susceptibility is not part of the prescribing process; there is no way of knowing what is doing what and how to proceed. There is no protocol involved only the vagueness of "tweaking" the drug regime either to manage side effects, or to help things improve.

This "polypharmacy", as it's called, has led to more hospital visits; over the past seven years, hospitals have had to deal with a 53% increase in serious side effects from this common "chemical cocktail".[6]

The third principle of homeopathy is to prescribe the minimum dose of the medicine, that is, the least amount of medical stimulation necessary to induce a change in a positive direction. The observation here, over several hundred years, is that once the self-regulating human organism has been stimulated to heal or recover the best thing is to allow it to do what it does best, to get out of its way and only re-prescribe if the recovery falters, or some complication occurs. In this homeopathic way, less is best and the best prescription is often nothing.

"To do nothing is sometimes a good remedy."

Hippocrates

In some cases, the minimum dose is a single pill, in others it can be one pill three times a day, or once a week. This minimum, or optimum dose cannot be guessed at but needs to be discovered through careful experiment and observation. As I tell each patient, "You are a one-off event in space and time and what is best for you is likely to be different to what is best for someone else."

This principle of the minimum dose resonates with the Arndt-Schultz law of Pharmacology, which states that: *"For every substance, small doses stimulate, moderate doses inhibit, large doses kill"*. This has been modernised and is now known as hormesis.

THE POTENCIES

When Hahnemann began to explore the effects of substances upon healthy people, he knew that some of them were deadly poisons; *Aconitum napellus* or Monkshood, for example. Thus, in the preparation of the doses he used a process of dilution (to minimize negative effects) followed by succussion, a vigorous shaking of the solution by repeated banging on a leather-bound book. The process of producing these "potencies", as he called them, is now carried out in well-regulated modern pharmacies all over the world, using machines for succussion.

A homeopathic potency then is a particular phenomenon, the result of serial dilution followed by succussion. A potency is not simply an "ultra-high dilution".

The substance to be prepared is macerated in alcohol and allowed to steep for a certain time. One drop of this solution is added to 99 drops of alcohol solution, and succussed. This is designated, 1C; one, one in a hundred dilution. One drop of this is then added to 99 drops of alcohol solution, and succussed. This is designated, 2C; two, one in a hundred dilutions. This process of dilution followed by succussion is repeated.

At 6C, six one in a hundred dilutions, this is the dilution equivalent of one drop of the original substance in several large swimming pools.

At 12C, which may also be written as 10^{-24}, Avogadro's constant (10^{-23}: the dilution beyond which no molecules of the original substance can remain) has been exceeded; this is the dilution equivalent of one drop in the Atlantic Ocean. From a material perspective this is clearly ridiculous. Well known scientists have said that, "it's like adding a drop of the medicine to the Atlantic Ocean in Ireland, flying over to America, taking a drop out of the sea and expecting your symptoms to get better!" That IS ridiculous, yet the process of serial dilution and succussion is categorically not the same as dropping any amount of solution into the Ocean, and actually involves just over a litre of alcohol solution. To assume that the end result of both processes is the same is just that, an assumption. No true scientist would make the basic mistake of assuming an outcome.

From a materialistic point of view homeopathy appears absurd; how can the medicine have any effect upon the patient if, as is generally, yet not always, the case, it contains no molecules of "active ingredient"? Part of the limitation of this point of view is that it continues to ignore one of the great truths that science has helped to elucidate, namely that the basic "stuff" of which the universe is made is energy; matter is only energy in its denser form. Ignoring this truth means to focus too much attention upon the material realm and to assume, for example, that molecules are necessary to stimulate a change in physiology. Upon what authority is it clearly stated that only a molecular stimulus can affect such a change? I challenge that authority. It is now the twenty-first century and time to bring "the new physics" into everyday thinking.

And, as that great hero of "the new physics" Einstein wrote:
"If at first the idea is not absurd, then there is no hope for it."

Commonly used potencies are 30C and 200C and patients commonly report improvement in symptoms when much higher potencies are prescribed. There is no limit to potency, which, surely, should make the phenomenon even more interesting to explore?

THE PROVINGS

A proving is the process through which the potential medicinal uses of a natural substance are discovered. Healthy human volunteers undergo a full homeopathic consultation and their current state of health is evaluated. They then participate in a double blind, placebo-controlled, randomised experiment in which the substance being tested is administered, in a range of different potencies. No participant has any idea what is being tested or whether he or she has taken the medicated or non-medicated tablets.

The 'provers' then carefully record all changes in their health, all changes in normal sensation and function. This includes any dreams of note, any moods, perceptions or persistent thoughts. Every day the prover speaks with an individually assigned supervisor whose task is to help clarify the information. Provers are forbidden to speak about their experience, to anyone. Only when symptoms cease is the proving over for that individual and, following a final conversation with the supervisor, the prover's journal is handed in to the proving coordinator. Collating all the information gathered in all the provers' journals and then arranging it systematically is a long and painstaking task. Nonetheless, the health of a patient may one day depend upon such accurate observation and recording.

In addition to the proving findings, information obtained by a close review of well-documented poison effects, as well as from clinical experience with the proved medicine, is gathered together and organized into the homeopathic Materia Medica. This consists of detailed information on over 2,000 medicines. To help find the correct medicine, information on symptoms - and which medicinal substance causes them - is organised into what is known as a Homeopathic Clinical Repertory. This is a kind of guidebook or index to the Materia Medica.

Proving accounts and the Materia Medica provide a vast store of medical knowledge and the homeopath spends a huge amount of time and energy studying them. The matching of patient symptoms to proving symptoms involves a methodical process that is part of the science of homeopathy.

Substances are tested for their medicinal potential on healthy people, not people who are already un-well and suffering. The provers ideally need to be articulate enough to describe the sometimes, subtle changes in their normal sensation and function. These are the changes which often precede tissue changes in the patient.

In my experience, all provers have experienced changes as a result of taking the substance, no matter what potency they engaged with. The only exceptions were those who took the un-medicated tablets. When the nature of the substance, and the symptoms which it induced, is revealed most provers are astounded that their personal experience was similar to that of the others; that it was as if they were one person. It is also comforting for the prover to know that their personal discomfort during the proving may, one day, be of help to patients.

THE PRACTICE

Most people who visit a homeopath have typically tried everything that modern medicine has to offer and are no better, or are worse because of adverse drug reactions. Most of these people have decided to try homeopathy because they know of someone who has benefited from treatment. There are no advertising campaigns.

The homeopathic consultation is a unique experience in medicine. In no other situation is the patient enabled to explore her/his health on every level, mental, emotional, physical, social or spiritual. This, of itself, can be a very empowering experience.

When I meet with a patient for the first time, it has become my practice to open our conversation in the following manner:

"My task is to listen to you, to observe you, to listen more deeply and to ask the right questions so that together we can explore what needs to change and, maybe, to get a sense of how you arrived at this position in your life. Then, I will try to find one or two homeopathic medicines which can, hopefully, help you to restore yourself to relative health. You will do all the healing; I will help and walk alongside you."

Listening, deeply listening, in an un-prejudiced manner, is central to homeopathic treatment. Through listening, and asking the questions which naturally arise from such listening, empathy is enhanced and the inner landscape of the patient's experience is carefully revealed.

Recent research has shown that when someone is describing an event they **had** witnessed, their brain patterning is similar to the patterning observed while they **were** witnessing. More interestingly, the brain patterning of an attendant listener becomes similar to that of the speaker.[7] Here is some evidence that "getting on the same wavelength" as someone else is demonstrable. This research also suggests that resonance and similarity are important factors in healing.

For the initial consultation with an adult I allow an hour and a half; for a child, one hour. This allows time to really explore the patient's experience of life and suffering. On one occasion, an open-minded GP sat in on my clinic and, after witnessing an initial consultation remarked: "That was extraordinary; it would probably take me eighteen months to get all that information, if the patient visited on a monthly basis".

The homeopathic consultation depends upon asking open questions, questions regarding sensations, feelings, thoughts, precise bodily locations, factors which influence the symptoms or behavior etc. "Please tell me how you experience that/ please tell me a little more about that/what is that like for you?" Important questions include, "when did your health change/what was happening in your life around that time?" The intention is to explore, and hopefully discover, what has disturbed the patient's health and how the patient is expressing that disturbance. Details of the patient's psychology, life story, personal and family medical history, reactions to environment, appetite, sleep patterns, menstrual history etc. complete the picture (it often takes several consultations to gather all this information).

The task then is to analyse all the information, decide upon the nature and possible cause of the diseased state and, most importantly, to choose the symptoms which are most individual to the patient. Example: itchy skin is a common symptom of eczema yet an itching which has a burning element to it and feels as if someone is stubbing out a cigarette, is unusual and is closer to the experience of the individual. The truly homeopathic medicine would be one which produced this symptom in a proving.

When the consultation process is complete my practice is to thank the patient for such an intimate sharing of their experiences. I then begin my response by saying: "I start from the position that I don't know anything; given that you are one of seven billion worlds on this planet, this seems to be the only reasonable position." I then report my observations and perceptions, checking that these resonate with the patient. I tell them what medicine I am prescribing, and the reason for it; again, I check that what I am suggesting makes sense to them. I ask if they have any questions and we have whatever conversation is required.

Homeopathic treatment is a process, a collaboration which takes place over time; follow-up consultations are essential for developing the return to health. Especially in the case of chronic disease, which has usually developed over some time, the prescription of several medicines is likely to be necessary, over time. Each follow-up involves a thorough investigation of any changes in health since the last consultation; this is vital to ascertain in which direction the patient is heading (towards health, or towards continuing sickness) and what to do next. There are no "side effects", only effects. The homeopath's task is to decide which are likely to be due to the action of the medicine (often a slight and temporary intensification of symptoms) and which are likely to be due to the reaction of the patient to the stimulus of the medicine (often enough, an improvement in symptoms). Whilst the action of a homoeopathic medicine is gentle, the reaction of the patient can be profound.

In my experience, the prescribed medicine either helps or nothing noticeable happens; there is either resonance with the patient, or not; it is either homeopathic to the case or not. Once again, this echoes the Hippocratic dictum: **"either help, or at least do no harm"**.

Many times, a patient has sent a card or a gift in appreciation of feeling much better following treatment: "You've cured my asthma/migraine/eczema etc." Whilst I appreciate the sentiment, it is my practice to suggest that practitioners never cure patients, patients cure themselves, with the help of the practitioner. Even following, for example, a brilliant surgical intervention to resolve a ruptured aortic aneurysm, the patient is taken to the recovery room where he or she recovers, or does not. Being a major part in their own return to health following illness is empowering for patients and encourages them to take greater responsibility for their health.

Every time I make a homeopathic prescription there are at least three factors at play; the placebo effect, the therapeutic relationship, and the medicine itself. I can never be entirely sure which is having the most effect at any one time. Apparently, "50% of the effectiveness of all drugs is due to the placebo effect".[8] Placebo is powerful medicine it seems yet I cannot really make use of this. I cannot make the patient believe in me or my medicine, something has to happen within them which I cannot influence, other than being authentically myself. The way in which I consult is unique to me, my nature and my experience and will resonate with the patient, or not. Most people in Western culture believe in modern mainstream medicine and so it is more likely that they will respond to any placebo effect through this kind of treatment than homeopathy.

Care, kindness and consideration can be enormously helpful of themselves.

"Cure sometimes, treat often, comfort always".

Hippocrates

Co-creating and maintaining a therapeutic relationship is a skill which requires endless practise, as every potentially therapeutic encounter is unique. Listening, observing and asking the right questions is the way to establish empathy, through which the practitioner gains a sense of the patient's experience and becomes, briefly, a similar sufferer. Empathy is the beginning of homeopathy.

A homeopathic consultation is often a very positive experience for a patient who may feel better in a number of ways afterwards. In my experience, any improvement in physical symptoms is generally short-lived unless the consultation is followed and supported by the prescription.

I know homeopathy works, when it seemingly does not. I have often prescribed once, twice or even three times before the patient will report significant improvement. This is evidence enough for me that the medicine has a definite effect if it is the one most homeopathic to the case. Selecting the best fitting medicine can be a lengthy and laborious process so if there was sound evidence that homeopathy only helps through the placebo effect then my work would be a lot easier.

What I continue to find extraordinary is how the homeopathic medicine can sometimes transform a patient's health completely or, if there is no positive change, no harm is done. Homeopathy is a completely safe form of holistic medicine. In over two hundred years of homeopathic treatment, all over the world, there has not been one recorded death directly attributed to the medicines.

HOW DOES IT WORK?

Homeopathy is effective. There is substantial significant evidence to support it plus the simple fact that around 600 million people in over 80 countries worldwide use it to get well and stay well.[9]

These people come from all walks of life and have simply made their own experience of homeopathy and found it to be helpful.

More research is required yet most medical research, and publishing, is controlled by the international pharmaceutical industry which is not able to patent potencies and, therefore, not able to make a lot of money. In addition, given the opprobrium conferred upon scientists who have supported the biological activity of potencies, it is not surprising that few would dare to challenge the scientific orthodoxy.

Even so, good science has produced several theories which might explain how a medicine containing no molecules of the original substance could exert a biological influence upon a living organism. It is beyond the remit of this little book to describe the science in detail but references are provided for those who wish to explore more fully.

1. Dr Iris Bell has researched and written extensively on how the science of nano particles might provide an explanation

for homeopathy; her experiments have been reproduced in laboratories around the world. Seemingly, nano particles (sub-microscopic in size) of the original substance remain within the potency past the 12th centesimal dilution, and have been demonstrated to influence biological activity within an organism, and upon cells grown in a petri dish.

Dr Bell works with the notion that, "human beings, animals, and plants are self-organizing, complex adaptive systems" which respond to the "information" communicated by the homeopathic medicine, which is "a complex, nano-scale system".[10]

2. Dr Alexander Tournier and Nobel laureate, Professor Luc Montagnier, describe how "coherence domains" might offer a quantum theory explanation. "High dilutions of something are not nothing. They are water structures which mimic the original molecules."[11]

3. Rustum Roy, a professor of Materials Science, Chemistry and Physics, with an illustrious 65-year career in science, suggested that the process of Epitaxy offers a possible explanation for how homeopathy works. Essentially, structural information from one substance, usually a solid, can be transferred to another substance, usually a liquid, with no exchange of material. This is applied in the micro-processing industry on a daily basis.[12]

What most theories suggest is that information pertaining to the original substance is transferred to water structures and, if the information resonates with the organizing principle of the patient, this triggers a response within the organism. It makes sense to me, and to patients, that the homeopathic tablet (which contains the potency) is akin to a CD with structural information of the original substance somehow imprinted upon it. Take two un-labelled CDs to any laboratory and ask for a chemical analysis and the result is likely to be: "Aside from a few impurities, they are identical". If the CDs were played, and the imprinted information were to be accessed, one might be a recording of a Mozart symphony and the other of a heavy metal band.

As self-regulating, self-creating organisms we exchange matter with our environment (food and water go in, waste products come out) and energy (heat, light, magnetic radiation) but most of all we are information exchangers and, to state the obvious, **information is neither matter nor energy, it pertains to pattern**.

Rupert Sheldrake, biologist and author, has written extensively about morphic resonance and the importance of similarity in Nature.

"Morphic fields are fields of probability, like quantum fields, and they work by imposing patterns on otherwise random events in the systems under their influence... (They) are inherited from previous similar organisms... (involving) a resonant transfer of form, or in-form-ation, from the past to the present... It works on the basis of similarity: the more similar, the more resonant."[13]

This echoes the simple hypothesis put forward by homeopathy: if the symptoms that a substance induces in healthy humans are very similar to those observed in the patient, then that substance will induce a positive change in the health of the patient. The more similar the symptom complex of the medicine to the symptom complex of the patient, the greater the resonance between the two. This hypothesis is proven over and over in daily practice all around the world.

EVIDENCE

There is sound evidence of homeopathy's effectiveness, in both acute, and particularly, chronic conditions. This evidence needs to be assessed by people who know how to do so, and who have no prejudice for or against homeopathy.

For example; by the end of 2019, 221 randomised controlled trials of homeopathy on 115 different medical conditions had been published in peer-reviewed journals. Of these, 129 were placebo-controlled on 77 medical conditions and were therefore eligible for detailed review.

- 45% were positive, finding that homeopathy was effective;
- 4% were negative, finding that homeopathy was ineffective;
- 51% were inconclusive.[14]

In addition, there have been six meta-analyses of homeopathy (large scale overviews of all previous research).

One meta-analysis was negative, concluding that homeopathy had no effect beyond placebo. Five were positive suggesting that there was evidence of an effect beyond placebo, but that more high-quality research would be needed to reach definitive conclusions. The most recent of these studies, published in 2014, found that homeopathic medicines, when prescribed during individualised treatment, are 1.5-2.0 times more likely to have a beneficial effect than placebo.[15] The team which carried out this research was led by Dr Mathie who concluded that it was an "unequivocally positive result for homeopathy".

In 2005, an observational study at the NHS funded Bristol Homeopathic Hospital included over 6,500 consecutive patients with over 23,000 attendances in a six-year period; 70% of follow up patients reported improved health, 50% reported major improvement. The largest improvements were reported in childhood eczema or asthma, and in inflammatory bowel disease, irritable bowel syndrome, menopausal problems and migraines.[16]

In 2008, a study in Germany followed over 3,500 chronically ill adults and children receiving routine homeopathic care from GPs over an eight-year period. At the start, 97% of participants were diagnosed with a chronic complaint with 95% declaring previous conventional treatment for their condition. The study found that, "patients who seek homeopathic treatment are likely to improve considerably" and that health benefits were steady and long term.[17]

There are more studies of this nature, especially from France, Germany and Switzerland-all countries where homeopathy is widely used.

In 2007, in Cuba, a dramatic reduction (84%) in the annual Leptospirosis infection rate was observed after the government, which was not able to produce vaccines for the entire population during an epidemic outbreak, gave a homeopathic medicine to 2.5 million people.[18]

With regards to the effectiveness of conventional medicine, things are not as clear cut as many people may believe. Every six months, the British Medical Journal (BMJ) publishes the scientific clinical evidence for treatments currently available on the NHS. This study found that of 3,000 commonly used NHS treatments 50% are of unknown effectiveness and only 11% are proven to be beneficial. See chart.[19]

SSRI anti-depressants, such as Prozac, are an example of such a treatment. These have now been confirmed as being no more effective than placebo in the treatment of mild and moderate depression, yet in 2006 the NHS spent around £150 million on them.[20]

The BMJ data clearly show that the NHS funds many treatments for which the evidence of effectiveness is unclear.

Effectiveness of NHS Treatments:

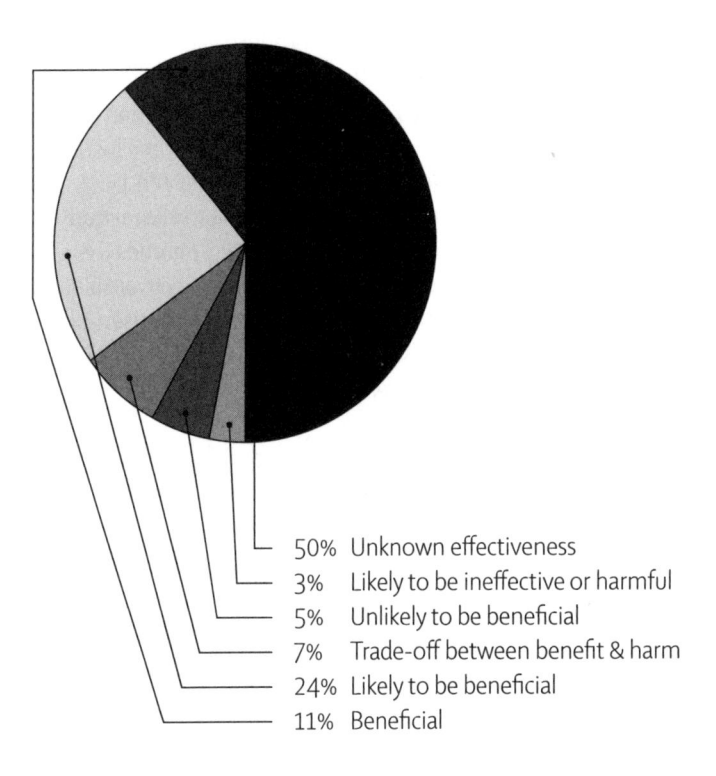

- 50% Unknown effectiveness
- 3% Likely to be ineffective or harmful
- 5% Unlikely to be beneficial
- 7% Trade-off between benefit & harm
- 24% Likely to be beneficial
- 11% Beneficial

BMJ Effectiveness of 3000 treatments as reported in RCT selected by Clinical Evidence.

SCIENTISTS

Many scientists, all over the world, have their own experience of homeopathy and concluded that there is good evidence for its effectiveness.

For example, Professor Jacques Benveniste, a doctor and allergy specialist, was research director at the French National Institute for Health and Medical Research during the 1980s. In 1985 one of his research assistants found some results that made no sense: a solution that had accidentally been diluted to the point where there was no possibility of any molecule remaining was found to have a biological effect. Benveniste, who had not even heard of homoeopathy, dismissed the result as an error but asked the technician to repeat the experiment. The same results were obtained.

Benveniste was a well-respected establishment scientist who came across something he could not explain...but he did not ignore it or cover it up. He pursued the research himself and produced sound and reproducible data demonstrating the biological effect of high dilutions. He coined the term 'the memory of water' to describe a possible mechanism for what he observed. Nature magazine, a prestigious scientific publication, infamously sent a team to investigate- and Benveniste became the focus of a scientific witch hunt.

His work was dismissed as a 'delusion', his professional competence, mental balance and scientific integrity questioned and his impressive reputation destroyed, seemingly by prejudice and poor science.

Other well-respected and experienced scientists have received similar treatment from the establishment, reviled in internet postings and dismissed as "friends of homoeopathy" or "homeopathic businessmen". They include Professor Luc Montagnier, a Nobel prize winner who wrote, "High dilutions of something are not nothing."[11] and Professor Rustum Roy, a Materials scientist who put forward Epitaxy as a possible explanation for homeopathy.[12] It seems absurd to suggest that well qualified scientists and doctors would have been charmed into a "system of quackery" without being significantly impressed by its effectiveness. This is especially so considering the social, economic and professional losses they would have incurred. The sneering, jeering and personal attacking by sceptics are symptoms of "astro-turfing"[21] in which misinformation is seeded at grass root level.

This kind of treatment harks back to Hahnemann himself who, at the age of sixty, was literally driven out of town by the apothecaries, ancestors of the pharmaceutical industry. This was essentially because he was getting better results than them and was challenging their complex and expensive prescriptions.

Around the same time, Ignaz Semmelweis, a Hungarian obstetrician, was ostracized by the medical community for having the temerity to suggest that doctors washed their hands after dissecting corpses and before then examining women in labour (puerperal fever was killing thousands of women after they had given birth, yet in his hospital the death rate was drastically reduced). It seems that scientific and medical orthodoxy rarely responds to challenge in an open and enquiring manner.

A decade after Benveniste's findings, Professor Madeline Ennis, well known for her scepticism around homeopathy, led a consortium of scientists to investigate the biological activity of highly dilute substances. In conclusion, she wrote: "Despite my reservations against the science of homeopathy, the results compel me to suspend my disbelief and to start searching for a rational explanation for our findings".[22] Such reservations are understandable; such re-searching would be helpful and, potentially exciting. However, who would risk their reputation to engage in such research, and who would be willing to fund it, given that any positive outcome would not be in the best interests of the international pharmaceutical industry?

Medical research is a costly and involved undertaking that is generally funded by large pharmaceutical companies, charities, trusts and governments. Millions of pounds are involved in drug development, which is usually recouped through licensing the drugs. As homeopathic medicines are derived from natural sources, they cannot be patented; without the financial returns that patents help to provide, it is more difficult to find companies willing to invest in homeopathic research. This is unfortunate, given that homeopathy has the potential to be a safe, effective and inexpensive complement to conventional health care.

Funding for research into other Complementary and Alternative Medicines has been steadily growing with promising results. Professor George Lewith (professor of Health Research at the University of Southampton) and others have received Government funding for their work.

The homeopathic profession encourages more research into homeopathy. However, the funding required for high quality research into homeopathy is not available in the UK at this time. Despite this the Homeopathy Research Institute (HRI) is an international charity created to address the need for high quality scientific research in homeopathy. In collaboration with the Carstens Foundation, the HRI website provides a clinical research database that contains over 1015 studies, from randomised controlled trials to observational studies. It is the most comprehensive and academically rigorous database of its kind in the world. [23]

In the current climate, where misinformation about homeopathy in the mainstream media is common, there is a need for clear communication of the facts about the evidence base for homeopathy. HRI therefore aims to provide decision-makers, academics, healthcare practitioners and patients with reliable, academically sound information about homeopathy research.

SCRUTINY

It is, of course, entirely reasonable that homeopathy, like any therapeutic modality, be subject to scrutiny, to have its *modus operandi* and evidence base challenged. It is entirely reasonable to be sceptical, to have an open mind and question things, in fact it is a requirement of common sense and good science. However, there is a fine line between scepticism and prejudice. Being sceptical means to have doubts: "I don't see how this can work". Being prejudiced suggests certainty: "This can't possibly work". In the 1950s, for example, many eminent surgeons were convinced that human heart transplants were impossible. As it turned out, they were wrong.

Because there are generally no molecules of active ingredient in the medicines, a frequently quoted criticism of homeopathy commences from the premise, therefore, that it cannot work. From a materialistic viewpoint this is an understandable position. It is also, however, a statement of prejudice, of pre-judgement. Given that a true scientist is an un-prejudiced observer, this position is also arguably un-scientific.

To the demonstrable fact that millions of people find homeopathy to be helpful, critics generally insist that this must be due to the placebo effect. However, this response risks closing down any meaningful research into both homeopathy and placebo. The effectiveness of placebo is evidence that molecules of active ingredient are not necessarily required. It is not reasonable to dismiss something simply because it is not understood.

In addition, the production of symptoms in a proving, as well as the frequently observed reaction of babies and animals[24] to homeopathic medicines, is unlikely to be due to any placebo effect. In 2010, The International Journal of Oncology published a paper demonstrating that four different homeopathic medicines, in various potencies, were shown to kill cancer cells yet not harm healthy ones; the experiments were carried out on cell lines cultivated within a laboratory[25] free from the likelihood of any placebo response.

To conclude that homeopathy is scientifically impossible because we don't know how it works seems to me to be unreasonable. It does, however, seem reasonable to conclude that it is scientifically implausible. This suggests a degree of open mindedness and the possibility of further research.

Charles Darwin was sceptical about homeopathy yet, after twelve years of continuous ill-health, he made his own experience and was treated by Dr Gulley, a homeopathic doctor, with very positive improvement. I suggest that a healthy scepticism involves the ability to hold a doubt at the same time as keeping an open mind.

Independent researcher Professor R. G. Hahn, Professor of anaesthesia & intensive care at Linköping University in Sweden and an internationally recognised expert in assessing medical research and meta-analyses, closely scrutinized the clinical trials on homeopathy and reached this verdict:

"To conclude that homeopathy lacks clinical effect, more than 90% of the available clinical trials had to be disregarded."[26]

HOMEOPATHS

According to the Institute for **Political, Economic and Social Studies Report of 2019 (EURISPES)** the global number of homeopathic prescribers is over 500,000 of which 50,000 are based in Europe.

Most of us were brought up in a materialistic culture and many of us were science or medicine trained. Most of us had never heard of homeopathy and if we had would probably have been sceptical of it. Like most people, we simply believed that if you were sick then you went to the doctor. Why then, did we change our minds?

The majority of us trained to be homeopaths as a result of some positive experience; of seeing it help a family member who was not responding to conventional medicine, or experiencing it ourselves. We wanted to know more about this medicine which shouldn't work, yet which clearly did work. To the scientific explorer in each of us, I suspect, this anomaly proved to be utterly irresistible.

Once you have seen a child screaming with earache, then take a little white pill and settle down to a peaceful sleep within a minute or so, there is no turning back; you have to know more about homeopathy. Once you yourself have experienced the transformative effects of a homeopathic medicine, you know that it works. Once you have practised for a few years and seen good results, you have to keep working.

You have to really want to be a homeopath. It is not easy. It is challenging to earn a modest living and challenging to bear the disrespect and ridicule of establishment medical science and the media. Yet the never diminishing privilege of helping people, seeing them get better, and their great appreciation of your work is more than a counter balance to any criticism.

"All truth passes through three stages. First, it is ridiculed. Second, it is violently opposed. Third, it is accepted as self-evident."

Schopenhauer

HOMEOPATHY

Homeopathy is a medical art. It is a synthesis of experience, philosophy and science grounded in careful observation over two hundred years and founded on principles which are easy to comprehend. Almost any condition which you might take to a GP could benefit from a homeopathic approach.

Homeopathy is a very safe form of medicine. Pregnant women, babies, senior citizens and people close to death have all benefitted markedly. The medicine either helps or at least does no harm.

Homeopathy is deeply ecological. Homeopathic pharmacies do not use chemical processes in the production of their medicines and only very small amounts of original material are needed. The use of natural resources then, is kept to a minimum and the medicines are inexpensive, of high quality, effective for many years and harmless to the environment when disposed of correctly.

Most homeopathic practices are independent and ethical small businesses. Most homeopaths are registered with a professional organisation, adhere to a code of ethics, and go about their work quietly; making no great claims for what they achieve they let their results speak for themselves. Big money is not being made, big advertising campaigns are not being mounted and fear is not being foisted on the public.

All people regardless of age, gender, ethnicity or ideology can benefit from homeopathy. Based as it is upon careful observation and experience, homeopathy can benefit people without any compromise of scientific or religious belief.

HOMEOPATHY AND THE NHS

Homeopathy has been part of the NHS since its inception in 1948 when the then government declared that homeopathy would continue to be available on the NHS as long as there were "patients wishing to receive it and doctors willing to provide it". Five homeopathic hospitals in London, Bristol, Liverpool, Tunbridge Wells and Glasgow were originally gifted to the NHS and, until 2017, treated around 40,000 patients every year. These patients had not been helped by mainstream medicine. Yet most responded well to homeopathic treatment.

In 2017, however, NHS England decided to end this service provision because they found "no clear or robust evidence to support the use of homeopathy on the NHS".[27] Only two homeopathic hospitals remain, in London and Glasgow. NHS England based its decision upon a number of research reports on homeopathy, most particularly that of the Australian National Health and Medical Research Council (NHMRC) and the UK Science and Technology Committee, Parliamentary Evidence Check.

The Australian NHMRC report, which was published in 2015, concluded that "the available evidence is not compelling and fails to demonstrate that homeopathy is an effective treatment". This contributed to world-wide damage of homeopathy's reputation. However, it was then discovered that there had been a report in 2012 which was much more positive about the effectiveness of homeopathic treatment; this report had been suppressed. The Australian NHMRC is now under investigation for bias and mis-reporting the evidence on homeopathy.[28]

The 2010 Parliamentary Evidence Check was produced by a small group of MPs but it is not a scientific document and should not be used or viewed as such. No systematic scientific method was applied, it was not carried out by experts in the field and the choice of evidence allowed into the consultation showed a notable bias. Such fundamental flaws have been widely acknowledged and 70 MPs expressed their concern about the entire process by signing an Early Day Motion (EDM908). In addition, an independent critique by Earl Baldwin of Bewdley concluded that the report was, "an unreliable source of evidence about homeopathy." Neither the Government nor the Department of Health acted on the recommendations of this report.[29]

So, neither of these two reports has any scientific validity and yet they have influenced NHS decision making and, unfairly and un-scientifically, damaged the credibility of homeopathy as well as deny NHS provision to thousands of patients.

How much money has been saved?
In 2016, the NHS cost the UK taxpayer over £127 billion[30]

with prescriptions alone amounting to £9.2 billion.[31] In the same year just £92,412 was spent on 40,000 homeopathy prescriptions.[32]

When considering value for money, it should be remembered that if these patients were not treated with homeopathic medicines, they would have to be treated by other NHS departments and either be prescribed the medicines which had not helped before, or have to take part in trials for new drugs, all of which would cost more than the homeopathic medicines yet with no guarantee of success. Financially and clinically, it is not a sensible decision. The only beneficiaries would be the drug companies.

Especially given that 50% of commonly used NHS treatments are of no known effectiveness (see Evidence) it would seem more sensible not to continue their provision; this would likely save several billion pounds.

Some years ago, an experienced GP sat in on my homeopathic clinic. There were a couple of new patients and a number of follow up consultations. I had particularly asked Claire (not her real name) to attend as I thought she might benefit from the GP's input. Claire had first come to see me some months previously in what she described as "a bad way". A year before this she had received a diagnosis of psoriasis on both feet, and been prescribed an oral steroid, steroid cream, and an antibiotic. Her whole body "just blew up", she developed allergic reactions she had never had before and fell into "a deep and heavy depression". Following homeopathic treatment, her allergies had disappeared and she was back to being the "sparky Mum" her family knew and loved. But whilst her feet were "much less bothersome", the psoriasis persisted.

At one point, towards the end of her consultation, with the GP examining her right foot and myself examining her left, Claire suddenly burst into tears and exclaimed; "Why can't I have this on the NHS?"

This might be more fully expressed as: Why can't we bring left and right brain approaches together?

Given that homeopathy is the second most used healing system in the world[33], has a good evidence base (see "Evidence"), is patient centred, safe and inexpensive, this seems a reasonable question. My strong suggestion is that the NHS seriously reviews the possibility of restoring the provision of homeopathy.

UNIFYING MEDICINE

We live in a constantly changing, dynamic and polarized universe; there is no certainty, no security. To insist that there is only one way to explore and make sense of things is unreasonable. There are over seven billion humans living on Earth, on this ball of rock and water falling through space; to insist that there is only one way to treat those who suffer with ill-health is also unreasonable, especially given the counter-experience of millions of those people. To insist upon either of these with certainty, is a movement towards dogma or fundamentalism, neither of which is helpful.

From a consideration of polarity, it may be suggested that mainstream medicine is essentially *logical, materialistic, objective, reductive, quantitative* and *masculine*; while homeopathy is more *intuitive, energetic, subjective, inclusive, qualitative* and *feminine*. They may be described as opposite poles of the same phenomenon; medicine. The mainstream approach is to prescribe medicines which act *against* the symptoms; the homeopathic approach prescribes medicines which act *with* the symptoms. My suggestion is that to insist on "*either/or*", one or the other, is narrow minded; that it is time, now, to be more whole-brained, to embrace holism with "*and/both*". It is my continued experience that many people would appreciate a broader vision of healthcare, a health service which is truly Hippocratic embracing both mainstream and homeopathic medicine.

The whole human world is becoming increasingly polarized by the divisiveness of "*this or that*". Everywhere is the tension between man and woman, black and white, rich and poor and the politics of left and right. I contend that if humanity is to mature then somehow, we need to embrace and make a space for all views and voices. I understand that this may not come easily. I encourage us all to try.

REFERENCES

1. www.nhs.uk/news/medication/almost-half-of-all-adults-take-prescription-drugs
2. digital.nhs.uk/news-and-events/news-archive/2017-news-archive/antidepressants-were-the-area-with-largest-increase-in-prescription-items-in-2016
3. "Deadly Medicines and Organised Crime: How Big Pharma has Corrupted Healthcare"; Dr Peter C. Gotszche; Taylor and Francis, 2013
4. www.theguardian.com/politics/2020/may/17/whod-be-a-health-secretary-five-former-incumbents-on-the-toughest-gig-in-politics
5. www.telegraph.co.uk/news/2017/11/15/half-over-65s-take-least-five-drugs-day/
6. www.wddty.com/news/2019/10/over-65s-taking-an-average-of-five-drugs-a-day.html#:
7. A.Zadbood, J. Chen, Y.C.Leong, K.A.Norman and U.Hasson, "How We Transmit Memories to Other Brains: Constructing Shared Neural Representations Via Communication", Cerebral Cortex 27, no.10 (2017):4988-5000, https://doi.org/10.1093/cercor/bhx202
8. www.livescience.com/42430-placebo-effect-half-of-drug-efficacy.html
9. EURISPES - The Institute for Political, Economic and Social Studies, Report 2019 - Use of homeopathy (all pg 62)
10. www.ncbi.nlm.nih.gov/pubmed/?term=Bell+IR)
11. www.homeopathy360.com/2017/01/21a-newquantumtheory

12. Rao ML, Roy R, Bell IR, Hoover R. The defining role of structure (including epitaxy) in the plausibility of homeopathy. Homeopathy. 2007 Jul;96(3):175-82.)
13. www.sheldrake.org
14. Faculty of Homeopathy, 2015. Research. Available from: facultyofhomeopathy.org/research/
15. Mathie RT, et al. Randomised placebo-controlled trials of individualised homeopathic treatment: systematic review and meta-analysis. Systematic Reviews, 2014; 3:142
16. Spence, D.S., Thompson, E.A. & Baron, S.J. (2005). Homeopathic Treatment for Chronic Disease: a Six-Year University-Hospital Outpatient Observational Study. Journal of Alternative and Complementary Medicine 11(5): 793-8.
17. Witt CM, et al. BMC Public Health, 2008; 8: 413.
18. Bracho, G, et al. (2010). Large-scale application of highly-diluted bacteria for Leptspirosis epidemic control. Homeopathy, 99(3): 156-66.
19. British Medical Journal (BMJ), 2015. What conclusions has Clinical Evidence drawn about what works, what doesn't based on randomised controlled trial evidence? Available from: clinicalevidence.bmj.com/x/set/static/cms/efficacy-categorisations.html
20. Kirsch I, et al. PLoS Med, 2008; 5(2): e45
21. Astroturf and manipulation of media messages", a TEDxUniversityof Nevada talk by Sharyl Attkisson
22. www.theguardian.com/science/2001/mar/15/technology2

23. www.hri-research.org/
24. Camerlink I, et al. Homeopathy, 2010; 99: 57–62.
25. P. Banerji et al.(2010). Cytotoxic effects of ultra-diluted remedies on breast cancer cells. International Journal of Oncology395-403, 2010
26. www.karger.com/Article/FullText/355916
27. www.england.nhs.uk/wp-content/uploads/2017/11/sps-homeopathy.pdf
28. www.hri-research.org/resources/homeopathy-the-debate/the-australian-report-on-homeopathy/
29. Bewdley, B., (2010). Observations on the report Evidence Check 2: Homeopathy by the House of Commons Science and Technology Committee. Retrieved from: ww.homeopathyevidencecheck.org/.
30. NHS costs: references required from Homeopathy Awareness
31. website
32. EURISPES - The Institute for Political, Economic and Social
33. Studies, Report 2019 - Use of homeopathy (all pg 62)

FURTHER READING

Hippocratic Writings,
Edited with an introduction by G.E.R. Lloyd; Penguin Classics, reprinted 1983.

Organon of the Medical Art
Edited and annotated Wenda Brewster O'Reilly Ph.D. based on a translation by Steven Decker: adapted from the sixth edition of the "Organon der Heilkunst" completed by Samuel Hahnemann in 1842. Birdcage Books, Palo Alto, California, 1996.

Einstein: His Life and Universe
Walter Isaacson; Simon and Schuster, 2007

Tao Te Ching
Lao Tsu; translated by Stephen Addiss and Stanley Lombardo; Hackett Publishing Company, 1993. *There are many translations, this one is a good place to start.*

ACKNOWLEDGEMENTS
HUGE THANKS TO:

The many hundreds of medical students from the University of Exeter School of Medicine and Dentistry, as well as the many hundreds of homeopathy students from all over the UK and Eire, who, in conversations over many years, intelligently challenged my explanations of homeopathy and so helped to refine and clarify my thinking and strengthen my desire to find common ground between mainstream and homeopathic medical practice.

Brian Turpin for skillful editing, perceptive comment, sound advice and good humour.

Mani Norland for sharing the vision and getting it out there.